The Effortless Guide to Mediterranean Meals

Super-Easy and Tasty Mediterranean Recipes to Save
Your Time and Boost Your Energy

Raphael Chapman

Table of contents

Delicious Chicken Tenders

Preparation Time: 10 minutes

Cooking Time: 15 minutes

Servings: 4

Ingredients:

- 1 1/2 lbs chicken tenders
- 2 tbsp. BBQ sauce, homemade & sugar-free
- 1 tbsp. olive oil
- 1 tsp. poultry seasoning
- Pepper
- Salt

Directions:

1. Add all ingredients except oil in a zip-lock bag. Seal bag and place in the fridge for 2 hours.
2. Heat oil in a pan over medium heat.
3. Place marinated chicken tenders on the hot pan and cook until lightly browned and cooked.
4. Serve and enjoy.

Nutrition:

Calories 366

Fat 15 g

Carbs 3 g

Protein 2 oz.

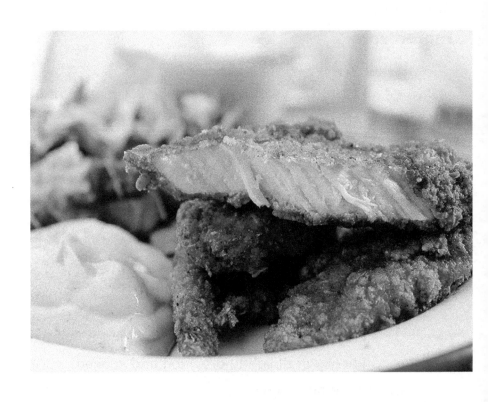

Grilled Pesto Chicken

Preparation Time: 10 minutes

Cooking Time: 10 minutes

Servings: 6

Ingredients:

- 1 1/2 lbs chicken breasts, skinless, boneless, and slice
- 1/4 cup pesto
- 1/2 cup mozzarella cheese, shredded
- Pepper
- Salt

Directions:

1. Place chicken into the large bowl.
2. Add pesto, pepper, and salt over chicken and coat well. Cover and place in the fridge for 2 hours.
3. Heat grill over medium-high heat.
4. Place marinated chicken on hot grill and cook until completely done.
5. Sprinkle cheese over chicken.
6. Serve and enjoy.

Nutrition:

Calories 300

Fat 14 g

Carbs 1 g

Protein 40 g

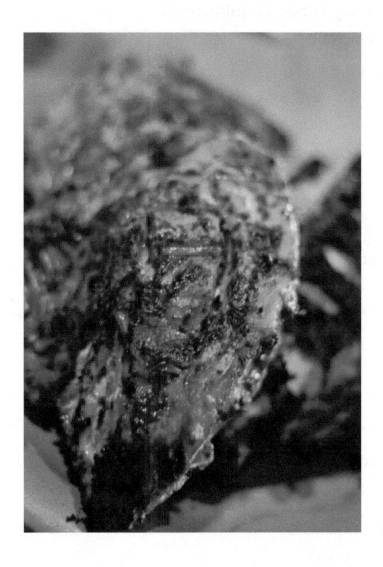

Easy & Tasty Salsa Chicken

Preparation Time: 10 minutes

Cooking Time: 2 hours

Servings: 6

Ingredients:

- 1 1/2 lbs chicken tenders, skinless
- 1/4 tsp. garlic powder
- 1/8 tsp. ground cumin
- 1/8 tsp. oregano
- 15 oz salsa
- 1/4 tsp. onion powder
- 1/4 tsp. chili powder
- Pepper
- Salt

Directions:

1. Place chicken tenders into the crockpot.
2. Pour remaining ingredients over chicken.
3. Cover and cook on high for 2 hours.
4. Shred the chicken using a fork and serve.

Nutrition:

Calories 235

Fat 8 g

Carbs 5 g

Protein 35 g

Tender Turkey Breast

Preparation Time: 10 minutes

Cooking Time: 4 hours

Servings: 8

Ingredients:

- 4 lbs turkey breast, bone-in
- 1/2 cup chicken stock
- 6 garlic cloves, peeled
- 3 fresh rosemary sprigs
- Pepper
- Salt

Directions:

1. Place turkey breast into the crockpot. Season with pepper and salt.
2. Add stock, garlic, and rosemary on top.
3. Cover and cook on low for 4 hours.
4. Serve and enjoy.

Nutrition:

Calories 235

Fat 3.5 g

Carbs 10 g

Protein 39 g

Chicken Bacon Salad

Preparation Time: 10 minutes

Cooking Time: 5 minutes

Servings: 3

Ingredients:

- 2 cups cooked chicken, shredded
- 1 cup cheddar cheese, shredded
- 1 cup celery, chopped
- 1/2 cup sour cream
- 1/4 cup mayonnaise
- 1/2 cup bacon, crumbles
- 3 green onions, sliced
- 1/4 cup onion, chopped
- Pepper
- Salt

Directions:

1. Add all ingredients into the large bowl and mix until well combined.
2. Serve and enjoy.

Nutrition:

Calories 482

Fat 31.3 g

Carbs 9.9 g

Protein 39.6 g

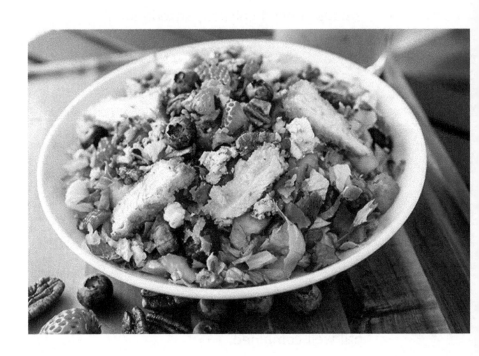

Green Salsa Chicken

Preparation Time: 10 minutes

Cooking Time: 3 hours

Servings: 6

Ingredients:

- 1 lb chicken breasts, skinless and boneless
- 15 oz green salsa
- Pepper
- Salt

Directions:

1. Add all ingredients into the crock pot.
2. Cover and cook on high for 3 hours.
3. Shred the chicken using fork.
4. Serve and enjoy.

Nutrition:

Calories 166

Fat 6 g

Carbs 3 g

Protein 22 g

Chicken Chili

Preparation Time: 10 minutes

Cooking Time: 6 hours

Servings: 4

Ingredients:

- 1 lb chicken breasts, skinless and boneless
- 14 oz can tomato, diced
- 2 cups of water
- 1 jalapeno pepper, chopped
- 1 poblano pepper, chopped
- 12 oz can green chilies
- 1/2 tsp. paprika
- 1/2 tsp. dried sage
- 1/2 tsp. cumin
- 1 tsp. dried oregano
- 1/2 cup dried chives
- 1 tsp. sea salt

Directions:

1. Add all ingredients into the crockpot and stir well.
2. Cover and cook on low for 6 hours.
3. Shred the chicken using a fork.
4. Stir well and serve.

Nutrition:

Calories 265

Fat 8.9 g

Carbs 11.1 g

Protein 34.9 g

Tasty Chicken Kabobs

Preparation Time: 10 minutes

Cooking Time: 10 minutes

Servings: 4

Ingredients:

- 1 1/2 lbs chicken breast, boneless & cut into 1-inch pieces
- 1 tsp. dried oregano
- 1 tbsp. fresh lime juice
- 1 tbsp. olive oil
- 1/2 tsp. pepper
- 1/2 tsp. sea salt

Directions:

1. Add chicken into the mixing bowl. Pour remaining ingredients over chicken and coat well and place it in the refrigerator overnight.
2. Heat grill over medium heat.
3. Thread marinated chicken onto the skewers.
4. Place chicken skewers onto the hot grill and cook for 8-10 minutes.
5. Serve and enjoy.

Nutrition:

Calories 228

Fat 7.8 g

Carbs 1.3 g

Protein 36.2 g

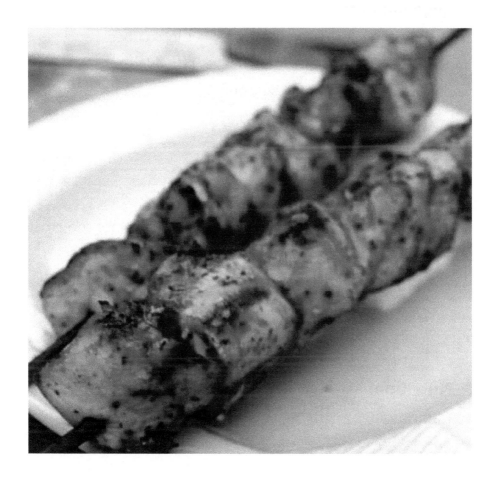

Cheesy Salsa Chicken

Preparation Time: 10 minutes

Cooking Time: 6 hours

Servings: 6

Ingredients:

- 2 lbs chicken breasts, cut into cubes
- 2 cups cheddar cheese, shredded
- 2 tbsp. taco seasoning
- 2 cups salsa
- Pepper
- Salt

Directions:

1. Add all ingredients except cheese into the crock pot.
2. Cover and cook on low for 5 hours 30 minutes.
3. Add cheese and stir well and cook for 30 minutes more.
4. Stir and serve.

Nutrition:

Calories 463

Fat 23.8 g

Carbs 5.9 g

Protein 54.5 g

Ranch Chicken Salad

Preparation Time: 10 minutes

Cooking Time: 5 minutes

Servings: 4

Ingredients:

- 3 cups cooked chicken, shredded
- 1/2 cup green onion, chopped
- 3/4 cup carrots, chopped
- 1 1/2 cups celery, chopped
- 1/2 cup mayonnaise
- 1/4 sweet onion, diced
- 1 tbsp. ranch seasoning
- 4 tbsp. hot sauce
- Pepper
- Salt

Directions:

1. In a small bowl, mix together hot sauce, ranch seasoning, and mayonnaise. Add remaining ingredients into the large bowl and mix well. Pour hot sauce mixture over salad and mix well. Serve and enjoy.

Nutrition:

Calories 275

Fat 13 g

Carbs 12 g

Protein 20 g

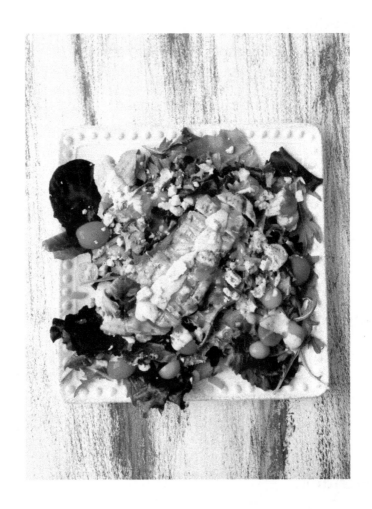

Harissa Chicken

Preparation Time: 10 minutes

Cooking Time: 4 hours

Servings: 4

Ingredients:

- 1 lb chicken breasts, skinless and boneless
- 1 cup harissa sauce
- 1/4 tsp. garlic powder
- 1/2 tsp. ground cumin
- 1/4 tsp. onion powder
- 1/2 tsp. kosher salt

Directions:

1. Season chicken with garlic powder, onion powder, cumin, and salt.
2. Place chicken into the crockpot. Pour harissa sauce over chicken.
3. Cover and cook on low for 4 hours.
4. Shred the chicken using a fork.
5. Serve and enjoy.

Nutrition:

Calories 230

Fat 10 g

Carbs 2 g

Protein 33 g

Almond Cranberry Chicken Salad

Preparation Time: 10 minutes

Cooking Time: 5 minutes

Servings: 4

Ingredients:

- 1 lb cooked chicken, shredded
- 1/4 tsp. garlic powder
- 1 celery stalk, chopped
- 1/4 cup almonds, sliced
- 1/4 cup cranberries, dried
- 1/4 cup mayonnaise
- 1/4 cup sour cream
- 1/4 tsp. onion powder
- 1/4 tsp. pepper
- 1/2 tsp. salt

Directions:

1. Add all ingredients into the mixing bowl and mix well.
2. Place in refrigerator for 1-2 hours.
3. Serve and enjoy.

Nutrition:

Calories 175

Fat 12 g

Carbs 6 g

Protein 8 g

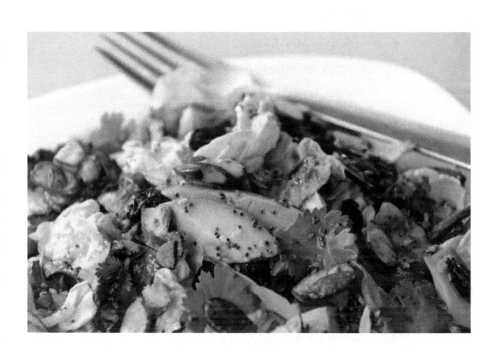

Simple Baked Chicken Breasts

Preparation Time: 10 minutes

Cooking Time: 45 minutes

Servings: 6

Ingredients:

- 6 chicken breasts, skinless and boneless
- 1/2 cup olive oil
- 1/4 cup soy sauce
- 1 tbsp. oregano
- 2 tbsp. fresh lemon juice
- 1 tsp. garlic salt

Directions:

1. Add all ingredients into the large zip-lock bag. Seal bag and shake well and place in the fridge for 3-4 hours.
2. Preheat the oven to 350 F.
3. Place marinated chicken into a baking dish and bake for 45 minutes.
4. Serve and enjoy.

Nutrition:

Calories 435

Fat 27 g

Carbs 2 g

Protein 43 g

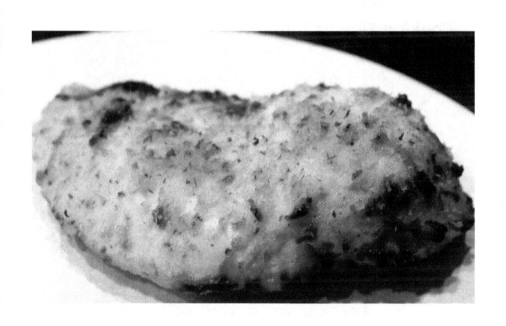

Baked Cod Fillets with Ghee Sauce

Preparation Time: 10 minutes

Cooking Time: 15 minutes

Servings: 2

Ingredients:

- Pepper and salt to taste
- 2 tbsp. minced parsley
- 1 lemon, sliced into ¼-inch thick circles
- 1 lemon, juiced and zested
- 4 garlic cloves, crushed, peeled, and minced
- ¼ cup melted ghee
- 4 Cod fillets

Directions:

1. Bring oven to 425o°F.
2. Mix parsley, lemon juice, lemon zest, garlic, and melted ghee in a small bowl. Mix well and then season with pepper and salt to taste.
3. Prepare a large baking dish by greasing it with cooking spray.
4. Evenly lay the cod fillets on the greased dish. Season generously with pepper and salt.
5. Pour the bowl of garlic-ghee sauce from step 2 on top of cod fillets. Top the cod fillets with the thinly sliced lemon.
6. Pop in the preheated oven and bake until flaky, around 13 to 15 minutes. Remove from oven, transfer to dishes, serve, and enjoy.

Nutrition:

Calories: 200;

Fat: 12g;

Protein: 21g;

Carbs: 2g

Avocado Peach Salsa on Grilled Swordfish

Preparation Time: 15 minutes

Cooking Time: 12 minutes

Servings: 2

Ingredients:

- 1 garlic clove, minced
- 1 lemon juice
- 1 tbsp. apple cider vinegar
- 1 tbsp. coconut oil
- 1 tsp. honey
- 2 swordfish fillets (around 4oz each)
- Pinch cayenne pepper
- Pinch of pepper and salt

Salsa Ingredients:

- ¼ red onion, finely chopped
- ½ cup cilantro, finely chopped
- 1 avocado, halved and diced
- 1 garlic clove, minced
- 2 peaches, seeded and diced
- Juice of 1 lime

- Salt to taste

Directions:

1. In a shallow dish, mix all swordfish marinade ingredients except fillet. Mix well then add fillets to marinate. Place in refrigerator for at least an hour.
2. Meanwhile create salsa by mixing all salsa ingredients in a medium bowl. Put in the refrigerator to cool.
3. Preheat grill and grill fish on medium fire after marinating until cooked around 4 minutes per side.
4. Place each cooked fillet on one serving plate, top with half of salsa, serve and enjoy.

Nutrition:

Calories: 416;

Carbs: 21g;

Protein: 30g;

Fat: 23.5g

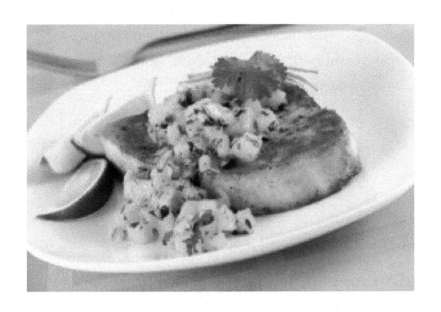

Breaded and Spiced Halibut

Preparation Time: 10 minutes

Cooking Time: 15 minutes

Servings: 4

Ingredients:

- ¼ cup chopped fresh chives
- ¼ cup chopped fresh dill
- ¼ tsp. ground black pepper
- ¾ cup panko breadcrumbs
- 1 tbsp. extra-virgin olive oil
- 1 tsp. finely grated lemon zest
- 1 tsp. sea salt
- 1/3 cup chopped fresh parsley
- 4 pieces of 6-oz halibut fillets

Directions:

1. Line a baking sheet with foil, grease with cooking spray and preheat oven to 400°F.

2. In a small bowl, mix black pepper, sea salt, lemon zest, olive oil, chives, dill, parsley and breadcrumbs. If needed add more salt to taste. Set aside.

3. Meanwhile, wash halibut fillets on cold tap water. Dry with paper towels and place on prepared baking sheet.

4. Generously spoon crumb mixture onto halibut fillets. Ensure that fillets are covered with crumb mixture. Press down on crumb mixture onto each fillet.

5. Pop into the oven and bake for 10-15 minutes or until fish is flaky and crumb topping are already lightly browned.

Nutrition:

Calories: 336.4;

Protein: 25.3g;

Fat: 25.3g;

Carbs: 4.1g

Berries and Grilled Calamari

Preparation Time: 10 minutes

Cooking Time: 5 minutes

Servings: 4

Ingredients:

- ¼ cup dried cranberries
- ¼ cup extra virgin olive oil
- ¼ cup olive oil
- ¼ cup sliced almonds
- ½ lemon, juiced
- ¾ cup blueberries
- 1 ½ lb. calamari tube, cleaned
- 1 granny smith apple, sliced thinly
- 1 tbsp. fresh lemon juice
- 2 tbsp. apple cider vinegar
- 6 cups fresh spinach
- Freshly grated pepper to taste
- Sea salt to taste

Directions:

1. In a small bowl, make the vinaigrette by mixing well the tbsp. of lemon juice, apple cider vinegar, and extra virgin olive oil. Season with pepper and salt to taste. Set aside.

2. Turn on the grill to medium fire and let the grates heat up for a minute or two.

3. In a large bowl, add olive oil and the calamari tube. Season calamari generously with pepper and salt.

4. Place seasoned and oiled calamari onto heated grate and grill until cooked or opaque. This is around two minutes per side.

5. As you wait for the calamari to cook, you can combine almonds, cranberries, blueberries, spinach, and the thinly sliced apple in a large salad bowl. Toss to mix.

6. Remove cooked calamari from grill and transfer on a chopping board. Cut into ¼-inch thick rings and throw into the salad bowl.

7. Drizzle with vinaigrette and toss well to coat salad.

8. Serve and enjoy!

Nutrition:

Calories: 567;

Fat: 24.5g;

Protein: 54.8g;

Carbs: 30.6g

Coconut Salsa on Chipotle Fish Tacos

Preparation Time: 10 minutes

Cooking Time: 10 minutes

Servings: 4

Ingredients:

- ¼ cup chopped fresh cilantro
- ½ cup seeded and finely chopped plum tomato
- 1 cup peeled and finely chopped mango
- 1 lime cut into wedges
- 1 tbsp. chipotle Chile powder
- 1 tbsp. safflower oil
- 1/3 cup finely chopped red onion
- 10 tbsp. fresh lime juice, divided
- 4 6-oz boneless, skinless cod fillets
- 5 tbsp. dried unsweetened shredded coconut
- 8 pcs of 6-inch tortillas, heated

Directions:

1. Whisk well Chile powder, oil, and 4 tbsp. lime juice in a glass baking dish. Add cod and marinate for 12 – 15 minutes. Turning once halfway through the marinating time.
2. Make the salsa by mixing coconut, 6 tbsp. lime juice, cilantro, onions, tomatoes and mangoes in a medium bowl. Set aside.
3. On high, heat a grill pan. Place cod and grill for four minutes per side turning only once.
4. Once cooked, slice cod into large flakes and evenly divide onto tortilla.
5. Evenly divide salsa on top of cod and serve with a side of lime wedges.

Nutrition:

Calories: 477;

Protein: 35.0g;

Fat: 12.4g;

Carbs: 57.4g

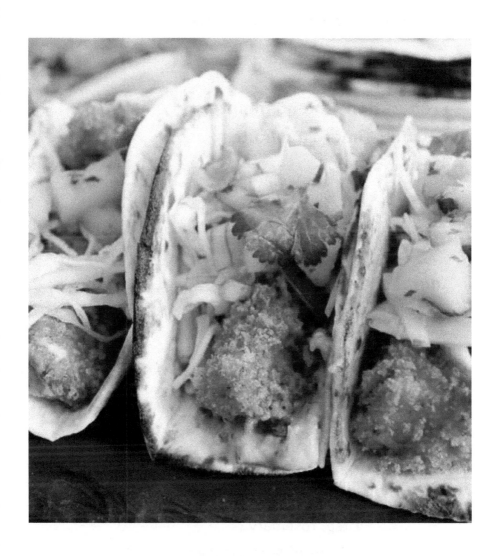

Baked Cod Crusted with Herbs

Preparation Time: 5 minutes

Cooking Time: 10 minutes

Servings: 4

Ingredients:

- ¼ cup honey
- ¼ tsp. salt
- ½ cup panko
- ½ tsp. pepper
- 1 tbsp. extra virgin olive oil
- 1 tbsp. lemon juice
- 1 tsp. dried basil
- 1 tsp. dried parsley
- 1 tsp. rosemary
- 4 pieces of 4-oz cod fillets

Directions:

1. With olive oil, grease a 9 x 13-inch baking pan and preheat oven to 375oF.
2. In a zip top bag mix panko, rosemary, salt, pepper, parsley and basil.
3. Evenly spread cod fillets in prepped dish and drizzle with lemon juice.
4. Then brush the fillets with honey on all sides. Discard remaining honey if any.
5. Then evenly divide the panko mixture on top of cod fillets.
6. Pop in the oven and bake for ten minutes or until fish is cooked.
7. Serve and enjoy.

Nutrition:

Calories: 137;

Protein: 5g;

Fat: 2g;

Carbs: 21g

Cajun Garlic Shrimp Noodle Bowl

Preparation Time: 10 minutes
Cooking Time: 15 minutes
Servings: 2

Ingredients:

- ½ tsp. salt
- 1 onion, sliced
- 1 red pepper, sliced
- 1 tbsp. butter
- 1 tsp. garlic granules
- 1 tsp. onion powder
- 1 tsp. paprika
- 2 large zucchinis, cut into noodle strips
- 20 jumbo shrimps, shells removed and deveined
- 3 cloves garlic, minced
- 3 tbsp. ghee
- A dash of cayenne pepper
- A dash of red pepper flakes

Directions:

1. Prepare the Cajun seasoning by mixing the onion powder, garlic granules, pepper flakes, cayenne pepper, paprika and salt. Toss in the shrimp to coat in the seasoning.
2. In a skillet, heat the ghee and sauté the garlic. Add in the red pepper and onions and continue sautéing for 4 minutes.
3. Add the Cajun shrimp and cook until opaque. Set aside.
4. In another pan, heat the butter and sauté the zucchini noodles for three minutes.
5. Assemble by the placing the Cajun shrimps on top of the zucchini noodles.

Nutrition:

Calories: 712;

Fat: 30.0g;

Protein: 97.8g;

Carbs: 20.2g

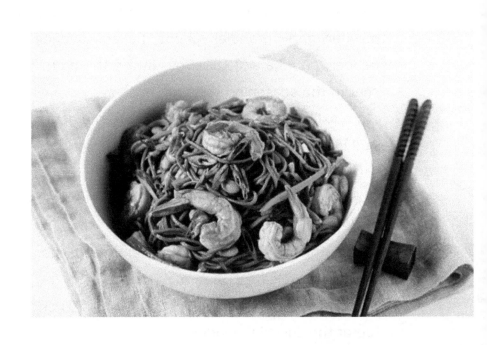

Crazy Saganaki Shrimp

Preparation Time: 10 minutes

Cooking Time: 10 minutes

Servings: 4

Ingredients:

- ¼ tsp. salt
- ½ cup Chardonnay
- ½ cup crumbled Greek feta cheese
- 1 medium bulb. fennel, cored and finely chopped
- 1 small Chile pepper, seeded and minced
- 1 tbsp. extra virgin olive oil
- 12 jumbo shrimps, peeled and deveined with tails left on
- 2 tbsp. lemon juice, divided
- 5 scallions sliced thinly
- Pepper to taste

Directions:

1. In medium bowl, mix salt, lemon juice and shrimp.
2. On medium fire, place a saganaki pan (or large nonstick saucepan) and heat oil.
3. Sauté Chile pepper, scallions, and fennel for 4 minutes or until starting to brown and is already soft.

4. Add wine and sauté for another minute.

5. Place shrimps on top of fennel, cover and cook for 4 minutes or until shrimps are pink.

6. Remove just the shrimp and transfer to a plate.

7. Add pepper, feta and 1 tbsp. lemon juice to pan and cook for a minute or until cheese begins to melt.

8. To serve, place cheese and fennel mixture on a serving plate and top with shrimps.

Nutrition:

Calories: 310;

Protein: 49.7g;

Fat: 6.8g;

Carbs: 8.4g

Creamy Bacon-Fish Chowder

Preparation Time: 10 minutes

Cooking Time: 30 minutes

Servings: 8

Ingredients:

- 1 1/2 lbs. cod
- 1 1/2 tsp. dried thyme
- 1 large onion, chopped
- 1 medium carrot, coarsely chopped
- 1 tbsp. butter, cut into small pieces
- 1 tsp. salt, divided
- 3 1/2 cups baking potato, peeled and cubed
- 3 slices uncooked bacon
- 3/4 tsp. freshly ground black pepper, divided
- 4 1/2 cups water
- 4 bay leaves
- 4 cups 2% reduced-fat milk

Directions:

1. In a large skillet, add the water and bay leaves and let it simmer. Add the fish. Cover and let it simmer some more until the flesh flakes easily with fork. Remove the fish from the skillet and cut into large pieces. Set aside the cooking liquid.

2. Place Dutch oven in medium heat and cook the bacon until crisp. Remove the bacon and reserve

the bacon drippings. Crush the bacon and set aside.

3.   Stir potato, onion and carrot in the pan with the bacon drippings, cook over medium heat for 10 minutes. Add the cooking liquid, bay leaves, 1/2 tsp. salt, 1/4 tsp. pepper and thyme, let it boil. Lower the heat and let simmer for 10 minutes. Add the milk and butter, simmer until the potatoes becomes tender, but do not boil. Add the fish, 1/2 tsp. salt, 1/2 tsp. pepper. Remove the bay leaves.

4.   Serve sprinkled with the crushed bacon.

Nutrition:

Calories: 400;

Carbs: 34.5g;

Protein: 20.8g;

Fat: 19.7g

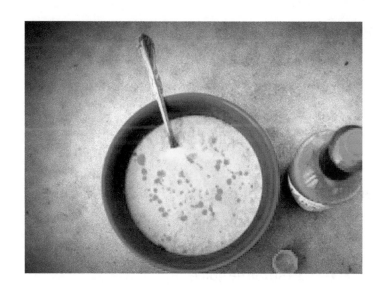

Crisped Coco-Shrimp with Mango Dip

Preparation Time: 10 minutes

Cooking Time: 20 minutes

Servings: 4

Ingredients:

- 1 cup shredded coconut
- 1 lb. raw shrimp, peeled and deveined
- 2 egg whites
- 4 tbsp. tapioca starch
- Pepper and salt to taste

Mango Dip Ingredients:

- 1 cup mango, chopped
- 1 jalapeño, thinly minced
- 1 tsp. lime juice
- 1/3 cup coconut milk
- 3 tsp. raw honey

Directions:

1. Preheat oven to 400°F.
2. Ready a pan with wire rack on top.
3. In a medium bowl, add tapioca starch and season with pepper and salt.
4. In a second medium bowl, add egg whites and whisk.
5. In a third medium bowl, add coconut.

6. To ready shrimps, dip first in tapioca starch, then egg whites, and then coconut. Place dredged shrimp on wire rack. Repeat until all shrimps are covered.

7. Pop shrimps in the oven and roast for 10 minutes per side.

8. Meanwhile make the dip by adding all ingredients in a blender. Puree until smooth and creamy. Transfer to a dipping bowl.

9. Once shrimps are golden brown, serve with mango dip.

Nutrition:

Calories: 294.2;

Protein: 26.6g;

Fat: 7g;

Carbs: 31.2g

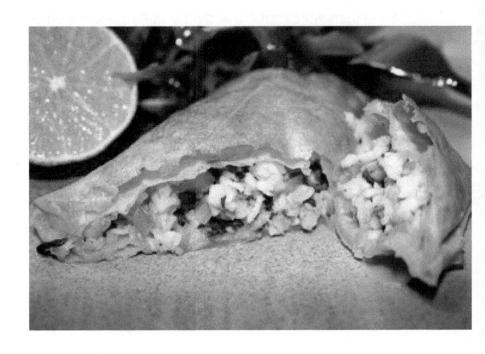

Cucumber-Basil Salsa on Halibut Pouches

Preparation Time: 10 minutes

Cooking Time: 17 minutes

Servings: 4

Ingredients:

- 1 lime, thinly sliced into 8 pieces
- 2 cups mustard greens, stems removed
- 2 tsp. olive oil
- 4 – 5 radishes trimmed and quartered
- 4 4-oz skinless halibut filets
- 4 large fresh basil leaves
- Cayenne pepper to taste – optional
- Pepper and salt to taste

Salsa Ingredients:

- 1 ½ cups diced cucumber
- 1 ½ finely chopped fresh basil leaves
- 2 tsp. fresh lime juice
- Pepper and salt to taste

Directions:

1. Preheat oven to 400°F.
2. Prepare parchment papers by making 4 pieces of 15 x 12-inch rectangles. Lengthwise, fold in half and unfold pieces on the table.
3. Season halibut fillets with pepper, salt and cayenne—if using cayenne.
4. Just to the right of the fold going lengthwise, place ½ cup of mustard greens. Add a basil leaf on center of mustard greens and topped with 1 lime slice. Around the greens, layer ¼ of the radishes. Drizzle with ½ tsp. of oil, season with pepper and salt. Top it with a slice of halibut fillet.
5. Just as you would make a calzone, fold parchment paper over your filling and crimp the edges of the parchment paper beginning from one end to the other end. To seal the end of the crimped parchment paper, pinch it.
6. Repeat process to remaining ingredients until you have 4 pieces of parchment papers filled with halibut and greens.

7. Place pouches in a baking pan and bake in the oven until halibut is flaky, around 15 to 17 minutes.

8. While waiting for halibut pouches to cook, make your salsa by mixing all salsa ingredients in a medium bowl.

9. Once halibut is cooked, remove from oven and make a tear on top. Be careful of the steam as it is very hot. Equally divide salsa and spoon ¼ of salsa on top of halibut through the slit you have created.

Nutrition:

Calories: 335.4;

Protein: 20.2g;

Fat: 16.3g;

Carbs: 22.1g

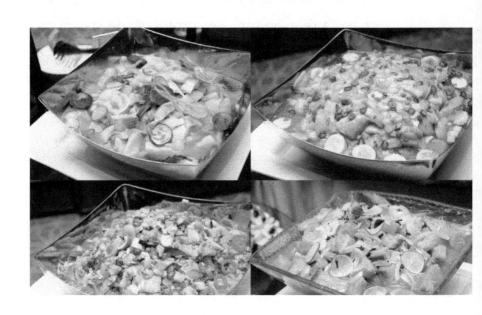

Curry Salmon with Mustard

Preparation Time: 10 minutes

Cooking Time: 8 minutes

Servings: 4

Ingredients:

- ¼ tsp. ground red pepper or chili powder
- ¼ tsp. ground turmeric
- ¼ tsp. salt
- 1 tsp. honey
- 1/8 tsp. garlic powder or 1 clove garlic minced
- 2 teaspoon. whole grain mustard
- 4 pcs 6-oz salmon fillets

Directions:

1. In a small bowl mix well salt, garlic powder, red pepper, turmeric, honey and mustard.
2. Preheat oven to broil and grease a baking dish with cooking spray.
3. Place salmon on baking dish with skin side down and spread evenly mustard mixture on top of salmon.
4. Pop in the oven and broil until flaky around 8 minutes.

Nutrition:

Calories: 324;

Fat: 18.9 g;

Protein: 34 g;

Carbs: 2.9 g

Dijon Mustard and Lime Marinated Shrimp

Preparation Time: 10 minutes

Cooking Time: 10 minutes

Servings: 8

Ingredients:

- ½ cup fresh lime juice, plus lime zest as garnish
- ½ cup rice vinegar
- ½ tsp. hot sauce
- 1 bay leaf
- 1 cup water
- 1 lb. uncooked shrimp, peeled and deveined
- 1 medium red onion, chopped
- 2 tbsp. capers
- 2 tbsp. Dijon mustard
- 3 whole cloves

Directions:

1. Mix hot sauce, mustard, capers, lime juice and onion in a shallow baking dish and set aside.
2. Bring to a boil in a large saucepan bay leaf, cloves, vinegar and water.
3. Once boiling, add shrimps and cook for a minute while stirring continuously.
4. Drain shrimps and pour shrimps into onion mixture.
5. For an hour, refrigerate while covered the shrimps.
6. Then serve shrimps cold and garnished with lime zest.

Nutrition:

Calories: 232.2;

Protein: 17.8g;

Fat: 3g;

Carbs: 15g

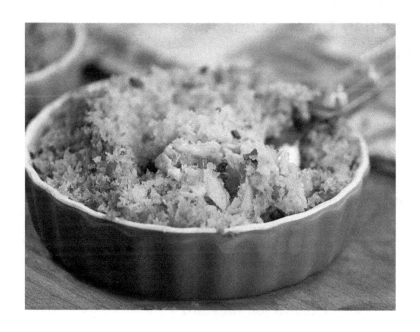

Dill Relish on White Sea Bass

Preparation Time: 10 minutes

Cooking Time: 12 minutes

Servings: 4

Ingredients:

- 1 ½ tbsp. chopped white onion
- 1 ½ tsp. chopped fresh dill
- 1 lemon, quartered
- 1 tsp. Dijon mustard
- 1 tsp. lemon juice
- 1 tsp. pickled baby capers, drained
- 4 pieces of 4-oz white sea bass fillets

Directions:

1. Preheat oven to 375°F.
2. Mix lemon juice, mustard, dill, capers and onions in a small bowl.
3. Prepare four aluminum foil squares and place 1 fillet per foil.
4. Squeeze a lemon wedge per fish.
5. Evenly divide into 4 the dill spread and drizzle over fillet.
6. Close the foil over the fish securely and pop in the oven.
7. Bake for 10 to 12 minutes or until fish is cooked through.
8. Remove from foil and transfer to a serving platter, serve and enjoy.

Nutrition:

Calories: 115;

Protein: 7g;

Fat: 1g;

Carbs: 12g

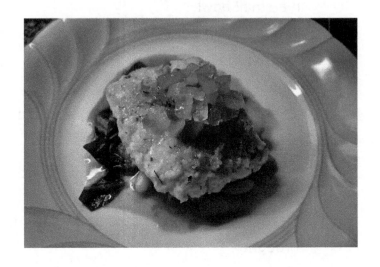

Garlic Roasted Shrimp with Zucchini Pasta

Preparation Time: 10 minutes

Cooking Time: 10 minutes

Servings: 2

Ingredients:

- 2 medium-sized zucchinis, cut into thin strips or spaghetti noodles
- Salt and pepper to taste
- 1 lemon, zested and juiced
- 2 garlic cloves, minced
- 2 tbsp. ghee, melted
- 2 tbsp. olive oil
- 8 oz. shrimps, cleaned and deveined

Directions:

1. Preheat the oven to 400°F.
2. In a mixing bowl, mix all ingredients except the zucchini noodles. Toss to coat the shrimp.
3. Bake for 10 minutes until the shrimps turn pink.
4. Add the zucchini pasta then toss.

Nutrition:

Calories: 299;

Fat: 23.2g;

Protein: 14.3g;

Carbs: 10.9g

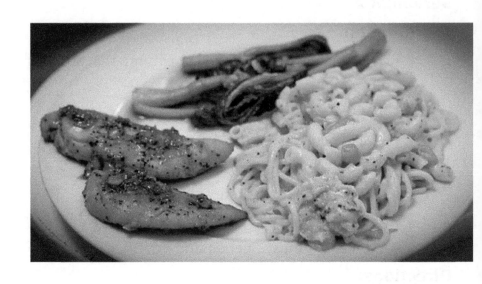

Jalapeno Lamb Patties

Preparation Time: 10 minutes

Cooking Time: 8 minutes

Servings: 4

Ingredients:

- 1 lb ground lamb
- 1 jalapeno pepper, minced
- 5 basil leaves, minced
- 10 mint leaves, minced
- ¼ cup fresh parsley, chopped
- 1 cup feta cheese, crumbled
- 1 tbsp. garlic, minced
- 1 tsp. dried oregano
- ¼ tsp. pepper
- ½ tsp. kosher salt

Directions:

1. Add all ingredients into the mixing bowl and mix until well combined.
2. Preheat the grill to 450°F.
3. Spray grill with cooking spray.

4. Make four equal shape patties from meat mixture and place on hot grill and cook for 3 minutes. Turn patties to another side and cook for 4 minutes.

5. Serve and enjoy.

Nutrition:

Calories 317

Fat 16 g

Carbs 3 g

Protein 37.5 g

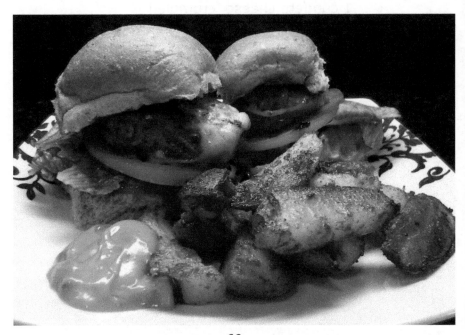

Basil Parmesan Pork Roast

Preparation Time: 10 minutes

Cooking Time: 6 hours

Servings: 8

Ingredients:

- 2 lbs lean pork roast, boneless
- 1 tbsp. parsley
- ½ cup parmesan cheese, grated
- 28 oz can tomatoes, diced
- 1 tsp. dried oregano
- 1 tsp. dried basil
- 1 tsp. garlic powder
- Pepper
- Salt

Directions:

1. Add the meat into the crock pot.
2. Mix together tomatoes, oregano, basil, garlic powder, parsley, cheese, pepper, and salt and pour over meat.
3. Cover and cook on low for 6 hours.
4. Serve and enjoy.

Nutrition:

Calories 294

Fat 11.6 g

Carbs 5 g

Protein 38 g

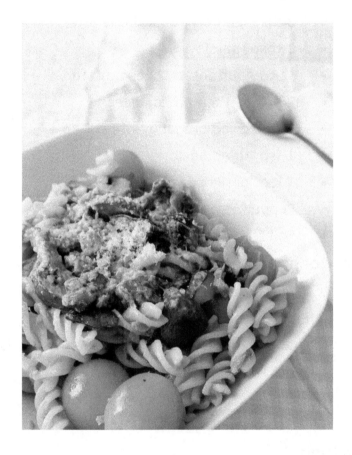

Sun-dried Tomato Chuck Roast

Preparation Time: 10 minutes

Cooking Time: 10 hours

Servings: 6

Ingredients:

- 2 lbs beef chuck roast
- ½ cup beef broth
- ¼ cup sun-dried tomatoes, chopped
- 25 garlic cloves, peeled
- ¼ cup olives, sliced
- 1 tsp. dried Italian seasoning, crushed
- 2 tbsp. balsamic vinegar

Directions:

1. Place meat into the crock pot.
2. Pour remaining ingredients over meat.
3. Cover and cook on low for 10 hours.
4. Shred the meat using fork.
5. Serve and enjoy.

Nutrition:

Calories 582

Fat 43 g

Carbs 5 g

Protein 40g

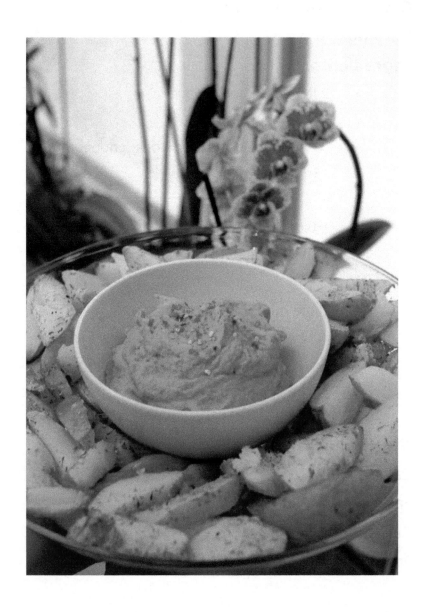

Lemon Lamb Leg

Preparation Time: 10 minutes

Cooking Time: 8 hours

Servings: 12

Ingredients:

- 4 lbs lamb leg, boneless and slice of Fat
- 1 tbsp. rosemary, crushed
- 1/4 cup water
- 1/4 cup lemon juice
- 1 tsp. black pepper
- 1/4 tsp. salt

Directions:

1. Place lamb into the crock pot.
2. Add remaining ingredients into the crock pot over the lamb.
3. Cover and cook on low for 8 hours.
4. Remove lamb from crock pot and sliced.
5. Serve and enjoy.

Nutrition:

Calories 275

Fat 10.2 g

Carbs 0.4 g

Protein 42 g

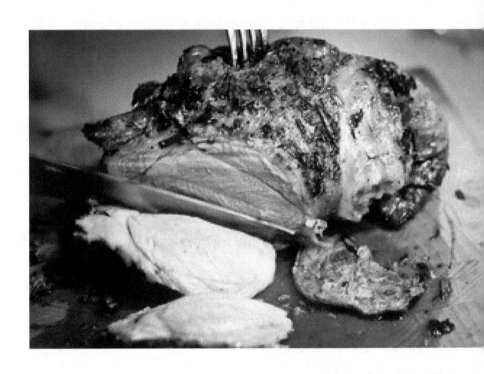

Lamb Stew

Preparation Time: 10 minutes

Cooking Time: 8 hours

Servings: 2

Ingredients:

- 1/2 lb lamb, boneless and cubed
- 1/4 cup green olives, sliced
- 2 tbsp. lemon juice
- 1/2 onion, chopped
- 2 garlic cloves, minced
- 2 fresh thyme sprigs
- 1/4 tsp. turmeric
- 1/2 tsp. pepper
- 1/4 tsp. salt

Directions:

1. Add all ingredients into the crock pot and stir well.
2. Cover and cook on low for 8 hours. Stir well and serve.

Nutrition:

Calories 297

Fat 20.3 g

Carbs 5.4 g

Protein 21 g

Flavorful Beef Stew

Preparation Time: 10 minutes

Cooking Time: 2 hours 5 minutes

Servings: 4

Ingredients:

- 2 lbs beef chuck, diced into chunks
- 3 thyme sprigs
- 2 bay leaves
- oz olives, pitted
- 3 cups red wine
- 2 garlic cloves, chopped
- 2 tbsp. olive oil
- Pepper
- Salt

Directions:

1. Season meat with pepper and salt.
2. Heat oil in a pan over high heat.
3. Add meat in hot oil and sear for 3-4 minutes on each side.
4. Add bay leaves, half red wine, garlic, and thyme. Bring to boil, turn heat to low and simmer for 90 minutes. Remove pan from heat.
5. Add olives and remaining red wine. Stir well.
6. Return pan on heat and simmer for 30 minutes more.
7. Serve hot and enjoy.

Nutrition:

Calories 630

Fat 20.3 g

Carbs 7 g

Protein 69.2 g

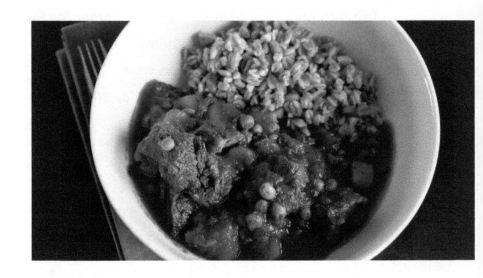

Herb Ground Beef

Preparation Time: 10 minutes

Cooking Time: 15 minutes

Servings: 4

Ingredients:

- 1 lb ground beef
- ½ tsp. dried parsley
- ½ tsp. dried basil
- ½ tsp. dried oregano
- 1 tsp. garlic, minced
- 1 tbsp. olive oil
- 1 tsp. pepper
- ¼ tsp. nutmeg
- ½ tsp. dried thyme
- ½ tsp. dried rosemary
- 1 tsp. salt

Directions:

1. Heat oil in a pan over medium heat.
2. Add ground meat to the pan and fry until cooked.
3. Add remaining ingredients and stir well.
4. Serve and enjoy.

Nutrition:

Calories 215

Fat 7.2 g

Carbs 1 g

Protein 34 g

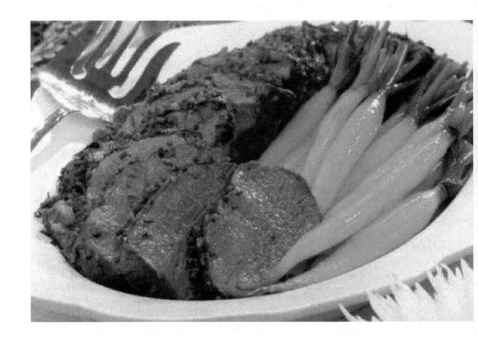

Olive Feta Beef

Preparation Time: 10 minutes

Cooking Time: 6 hours

Servings: 8

Ingredients:

- 2 lbs beef stew meat, cut into half-inch pieces
- 1 cup olives, pitted and cut in half
- 30 oz can tomatoes, diced
- 1/2 cup feta cheese, crumbled
- 1/4 tsp. pepper
- 1/2 tsp. salt

Directions:

1. Add all ingredients into the crock pot and stir well.
2. Cover and cook on high for 6 hours.
3. Season with pepper and salt.
4. Stir well and serve.

Nutrition:

Calories 370

Fat 14 g

Carbs 9 g

Protein 49.1 g

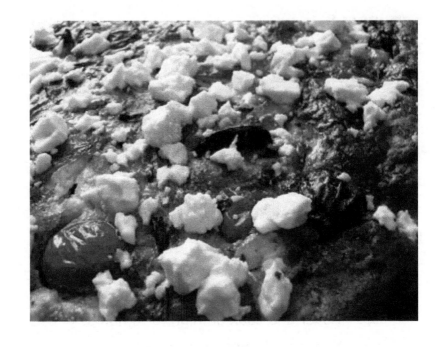

Italian Beef Casserole

Preparation Time: 10 minutes

Cooking Time: 1 hour 30 minutes

Servings: 6

Ingredients:

- 1 lb lean stew beef, cut into chunks
- 3 tsp. paprika
- 4 oz black olives, sliced
- 7 oz can tomatoes, chopped
- 1 tbsp. tomato puree
- 1/4 tsp. garlic powder
- 2 tsp. herb de Provence
- 2 cups beef stock
- 2 tbsp. olive oil

Directions:

1. Preheat the oven to 350°F.
2. Heat oil in a pan over medium heat.
3. Add meat to the pan and cook until brown.
4. Add stock, olives, tomatoes, tomato puree, garlic powder, herb de Provence, and paprika. Stir well and bring to boil.
5. Transfer meat mixture to the casserole dish.
6. Cover and cook in preheated oven for 1 1/2 hours.

7. Serve and enjoy.

Nutrition:

Calories 228

Fat 11.6 g

Carbs 6 g

Protein 26 g

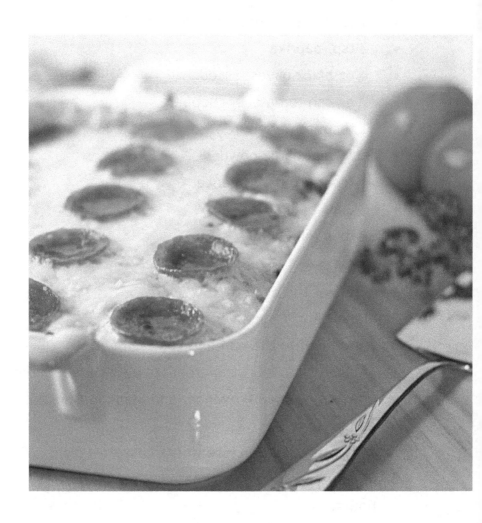

Roasted Sirloin Steak

Preparation Time: 10 minutes

Cooking Time: 30 minutes

Servings: 6

Ingredients:

- 2 lbs sirloin steak, cut into 1" cubes
- 2 garlic cloves, minced
- 3 tbsp. fresh lemon juice
- 1 tsp. dried oregano
- 1/4 cup water
- 1/4 cup olive oil
- 2 cups fresh parsley, chopped
- 1/2 tsp. pepper
- 1 tsp. salt

Directions:

1. Add all ingredients except beef into the large bowl and mix well.
2. Pour bowl mixture into the large zip-lock bag.
3. Add beef to the bag and shake well and refrigerate for 1 hour.
4. Preheat the oven 400°F.
5. Place marinated beef on a baking tray and bake in preheated oven for 30 minutes.
6. Serve and enjoy.

Nutrition:

Calories 365

Fat 18.1 g

Carbs 2 g

Protein 46.6 g

Easy Pork Kabobs

Preparation Time: 10 minutes

Cooking Time: 4 hours 20 minutes

Servings: 6

Ingredients:

- 2 lbs pork tenderloin, cut into 1-inch cubes
- 1 onion, chopped
- ½ cup olive oil
- ½ cup red wine vinegar
- 2 tbsp. fresh parsley, chopped
- 2 garlic cloves, chopped
- Pepper
- Salt

Directions:

1. In a large zip-lock bag, mix together red wine vinegar, parsley, garlic, onion, and oil.
2. Add meat to bag and marinate in the refrigerator for overnight.
3. Remove marinated pork from refrigerator and thread onto soaked wooden skewers. Season with pepper and salt.
4. Preheat the grill over high heat.
5. Grill pork for 3-4 minutes on each side.
6. Serve and enjoy.

Nutrition:

Calories 375

Fat 22 g

Carbs 7.5 g

Protein 58.5 g

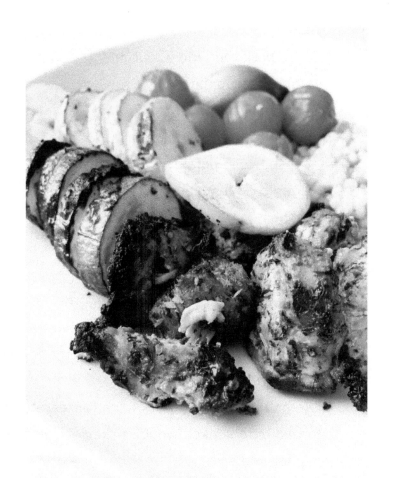

Meatballs

Preparation Time: 10 minutes

Cooking Time: 4 hours

Servings: 6

Ingredients:

- 1 egg
- 2 tbsp. fresh parsley, chopped
- 1 garlic clove, minced
- ½ lb ground beef
- ½ lb ground pork
- 14 oz can tomatoes, crushed
- 2 tbsp. fresh basil, chopped
- ¼ tsp. pepper
- ½ tsp. salt

Directions:

1. In a mixing bowl, mix together beef, pork, egg, parsley, garlic, pepper, and salt until well combined.
2. Make small balls from meat mixture.
3. Arrange meatballs into the slow cooker.
4. Pour crushed tomatoes, basil, pepper, and salt over meatballs.
5. Cover and cook on low for 4 hours.
6. Serve and enjoy.

Nutrition:

Calories 150

Fat 4 g

Carbs 4 g

Protein 24 g

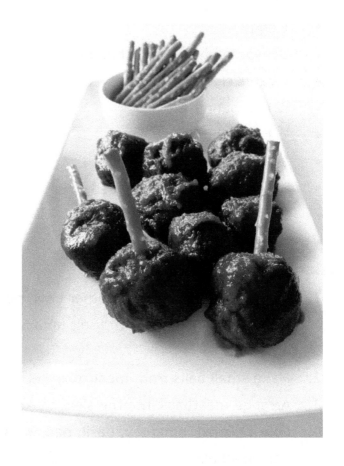

Baked Patties

Preparation Time: 10 minutes

Cooking Time: 15 minutes

Servings: 4

Ingredients:

- 1 lb ground lamb
- 1 tsp. ground coriander
- 1 tsp. ground cumin
- ¼ cup fresh parsley, chopped
- ¼ cup onion, minced
- ¼ tsp. cayenne pepper
- ½ tsp. ground allspice
- 1 tsp. ground cinnamon
- 1 tbsp. garlic, minced
- ¼ tsp. pepper
- 1 tsp. kosher salt

Directions:

1. Preheat the oven to 450°F.
2. Add all ingredients into the large bowl and mix until well combined.
3. Make small balls from meat mixture and place on a baking tray and lightly flatten the meatballs with back on spoon.
4. Bake in preheated oven for 12-15 minutes.
5. Serve and enjoy.

Nutrition:

Calories 112

Fat 4.3 g

Carbs 1.3 g

Protein 16 g

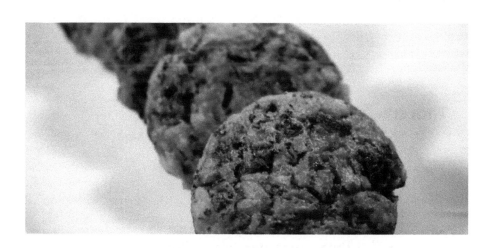

Keto Beef Patties

Preparation Time: 10 minutes

Cooking Time: 8 minutes

Servings: 5

Ingredients:

- 1 lb ground beef
- 1 egg, lightly beaten
- 3 tbsp. almond flour
- 1 small onion, grated
- 2 tbsp. fresh parsley, chopped
- 1 tsp. dry oregano
- 1 tsp. dry mint
- Pepper
- Salt

Directions:

1. Add all ingredients into the mixing bowl and mix until combined.
2.   Make small patties from the meat mixture.
3. Heat grill pan over medium-high heat.
4. Place patties in a hot pan and cook for 4-5 minutes on each side.
5. Serve and enjoy.

Nutrition:

Calories 188

Fat 6.6 g

Carbs 1.7 g

Protein 28.9 g

Tender & Juicy Lamb Roast

Preparation Time: 10 minutes

Cooking Time: 8 hours

Servings: 8

Ingredients:

- 4 lbs lamb roast, boneless
- ½ tsp. thyme
- 1 tsp. oregano
- 4 garlic cloves, cut into slivers
- ½ tsp. marjoram
- ¼ tsp. pepper
- 2 tsp. salt

Directions:

1. Using a sharp knife make small cuts all over meat then insert garlic slivers into the cuts.

2. In a small bowl, mix together marjoram, thyme, oregano, pepper, and salt and rub all over lamb roast.
3. Place lamb roast into the slow cooker.
4. Cover and cook on low for 8 hours.
5. Serve and enjoy.

Nutrition:

Calories 605

Fat 48 g

Carbs 0.7 g

Protein 36 g

Basil Cheese Pork Roast

Preparation Time: 10 minutes

Cooking Time: 6 hours

Servings: 8

Ingredients:

- 2 lbs lean pork roast, boneless
- 1 tsp. garlic powder
- 1 tbsp. parsley
- ½ cup cheddar cheese, grated
- 30 oz can tomatoes, diced
- 1 tsp. dried oregano
- 1 tsp. dried basil
- Pepper
- Salt

Directions:

1. Add the meat into the crock pot.
2. Mix together tomatoes, oregano, basil, garlic powder, parsley, cheese, pepper, and salt and pour over meat.
3. Cover and cook on low for 6 hours.
4. Serve and enjoy.

Nutrition:

Calories 260

Fat 9 g

Carbs 5.5 g

Protein 35 g

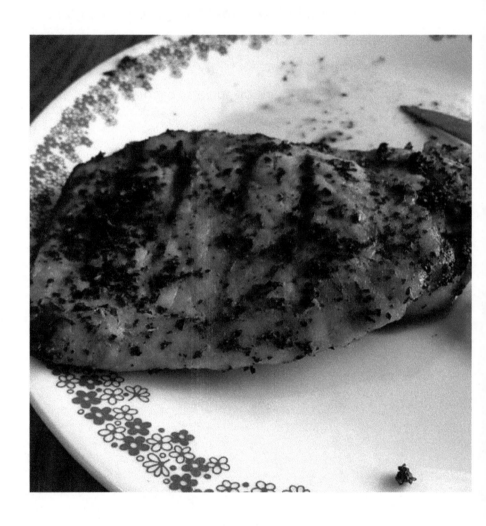

Feta Lamb Patties

Preparation Time: 10 minutes

Cooking Time: 12 minutes

Servings: 4

Ingredients:

- 1 lb ground lamb
- 1/2 tsp. garlic powder
- 1/2 cup feta cheese, crumbled
- 1/4 cup mint leaves, chopped
- 1/4 cup roasted red pepper, chopped
- 1/4 cup onion, chopped
- Pepper
- Salt

Directions:

1. Add all ingredients into the bowl and mix until well combined.
2. Spray pan with cooking spray and heat over medium-high heat.
3. Make small patties from meat mixture and place on hot pan and cook for 6-7 minutes on each side.
4. Serve and enjoy.

Nutrition:

Calories 270

Fat 12 g

Carbs 2.9 g

Protein 34.9 g

BBQ Pulled Chicken

Preparation Time: 10 minutes

Cooking Time: 45 minutes

Servings: 6

Ingredients:

- 1.5-lb. chicken breast, skinless, boneless
- 2 tbsp. BBQ sauce
- 1 tbsp. butter
- 1 tsp. Dijon mustard
- 1 tbsp. olive oil
- 1 tsp. cream cheese
- 1 tsp. salt
- 1 tsp. cayenne pepper

Directions:

1. Sprinkle the chicken breast with cayenne pepper, salt, and olive oil.
2. Place it in the baking tray and bake for 35 minutes at 365°F. Flip it from time to time to avoid burning.
3. When the chicken breast is cooked, transfer it on the chopping board and shred with the help of the fork.
4. Put the shredded chicken in the saucepan.
5. Add butter, cream cheese, mustard, and BBQ sauce. Mix up gently and heat it up until boiling.
6. Remove the cooked meal from the heat and stir well.

Nutrition:

Calories 154,

Fat 7.3 g,

Carbs 2 g,

Protein 24.4 g

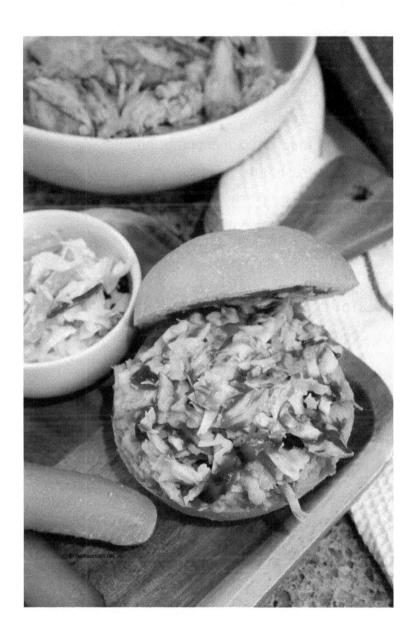

Flavorful Lemon Chicken Tacos

Preparation Time: 10 minutes

Cooking Time: 4 hours

Servings: 8

Ingredients:

- 2 lbs chicken breasts, boneless
- oz salsa
- 1 tbsp. taco seasoning, homemade
- 2 fresh lime juice
- 1/4 cup fresh parsley, chopped
- 1/4 tsp. red chili powder
- Pepper
- Salt

Directions:

1. Place chicken into the crockpot.
2. Pour ingredients over the chicken.
3. Cover and cook on high for 4 hours.
4. Shred the chicken using a fork and serve.

Nutrition:

Calories 235

Fat 8 g

Carbs 5 g

Protein 30 g

Crisp Chicken Carnitas

Preparation Time: 10 minutes

Cooking Time: 4 hours

Servings: 8

Ingredients:

- 2 lbs chicken breasts, skinless and boneless
- 1/4 cup fresh parsley, chopped
- 1 tbsp. garlic, minced
- 2 tsp. cumin powder
- 2 tbsp. fresh lime juice
- 1 tbsp. chili powder
- 1/2 tsp. salt

Directions:

1. Add chicken into the crockpot.
2. Pour remaining ingredients over the chicken.
3. Cover and cook on high for 4 hours.
4. Shred the chicken using a fork.
5. Transfer shredded chicken on a baking tray and broil for 5 minutes.
6. Serve and enjoy.

Nutrition:

Calories 225

Fat 8.7 g

Carbs 2.1 g

Protein 33.2 g

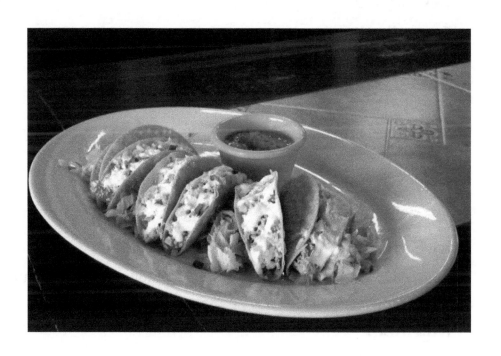

Cilantro Lime Chicken Salad

Preparation Time: 10 minutes

Cooking Time: 5 minutes

Servings: 2

Ingredients:

- 1 1/2 cups cooked chicken, shredded
- 2 tbsp. fresh lime juice
- 2 tbsp. fresh cilantro, chopped
- 2 tbsp. green onion, sliced
- 1 tsp. chili powder
- Pepper
- Salt

Directions:

1. Add all ingredients into the medium bowl and mix well. Season with pepper and salt.

Nutrition:

Calories 113

Fat 2 g

Carbs 1 g

Protein 20 g

Shredded Turkey Breast

Preparation Time: 10 minutes

Cooking Time: 8 hours

Servings: 10

Ingredients:

- 4 lbs turkey breast, skinless, boneless, and halves
- 1 1/2 tbsp. taco seasoning, homemade
- 12 oz chicken stock
- 1/2 cup butter, cubed
- Pepper
- Salt

Directions:

1. Place turkey breast into the crockpot.
2. Pour remaining ingredients over turkey breast.
3. Cover and cook on low for 8 hours.
4. Shred turkey breast with a fork.
5. Serve and enjoy.

Nutrition:

Calories 327

Fat 15.4 g

Carbs 11.8 g

Protein 34.3 g

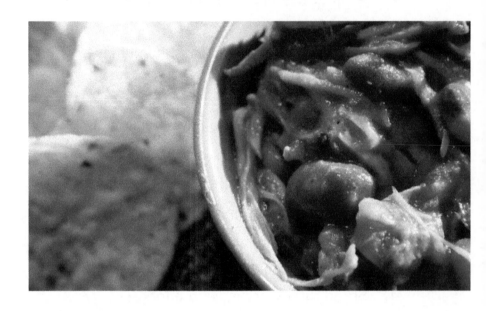

9 781802 693966